Introduction

The abbreviation OMAD has become pervasive and is before long acquiring such a lot of prominence in the field of time-limited fasting. You may have been considering what your companions mean when they allude to the OMAD diet. You are in good company! You are on the right course.

OMAD diet is certifiably not another turn of events; the main wind in it is that it is a well time-arranged slimming down system. There are recorded confirmations that let us know that antiquated Romans eat one time each day, which is typically a huge supper. What time they decided to eat, we can't actually tell.

Recently, a few superstars have come out to depict OMAD as a powerful weight reduction technique, just as a method for combatting persistent sickness and other wellbeing complications.

Some follow this eating design for strict reasons; in the mean time, some do it for transient weight reduction plan, while it has turned into a lifestyle for a few. It is simple that the OMAD diet isn't appropriate for everybody. Who are they? Perusing further will assist you with finding out.

'My companion does OMAD diet plan, so I should check it out", this assertion experiences put so many in difficulty. As powerful as the OMAD diet plan is, it has negative aftereffects in certain people, and it is exceptionally dangerous for some.

In this work, you see whether the OMAD diet plan could be appropriate for you, the advantages you remain to acquire from the eating-confining arrangement, and how you can accomplish the best outcomes. Then again, you will be presented to the wellbeing hazard of the OMAD diet plan, just as knowing whether it is ideal for you. What happens when you practice the OMAD diet in the long-term? How do I know I am not fit for the OMAD diet? Is it ideal for losing weight only? These questions and many more questions are well addressed based on personal and clinical experience.

What is the OMAD Diet?

◆ ◆ ◆

The abbreviation OMAD just means One Meal A Day.

O-One

M-Meal

A - A

D - Diet

What does this tell you? This eating regimen permits you to quick for 23 hours of the day, while permitted to eat inside an hour taking care of period. Sticking to the OMAD diet, the calories of food taken during the taking care of window period is equivalent to your day by day calorie admission. You know why? You are permitted to eat once in 24 hours inside the one-hour eating window after that hour has passed, you are not permitted to eat until the following 23 hours.

<u>A common example:</u>

Mrs. Agnes was told to participate in the OMAD diet plan for an underlying time of 14 days. She began the fifth of May by gobbling a dinner at 16:00 up till 17:00. Keeping the rule of the OMAD diet, what time is she expected to have her next meal?

You don't need to do quite a bit of arithmetic to know when next Mrs. Agnes will have her next supper. Her next taking care of period will be on the sixth of May at 16:00. She is relied upon to break her quick whenever from 16:00 and shouldn't eat pass 16:59. In any case, she is allowed to eat however much she can take inside the eating window period.

Mind you, one of the guidelines of the OMAD diet is consistency-You need to take and hold fast stringently to time.

The OMAD diet doesn't indicate what sort of food you ought to burn-through during the time of taking care of neither how much calories you ought to burn-through. Be that as it may, you should try to take care of inside your day by day calorie target.

OMAD vs. intermittent fasting

There is no contest between the two terms, the One Meal A Day (OMAD) diet is a variation of the discontinuous fasting. OMAD diet is an outrageous adaptation of time-limited eating, very much like discontinuous fasting. They look quite similar, right? Yes! But here is the difference:

While the discontinuous fasting provides you with the honor of a four or eight-hour eating window, the OMAD diet confines you to an eating-window of simply an hour and afterward quick for the other 23 hours of the day.

Enormous enough distinction, isn't that so? Yes!

Why some health practitioners don't recommend OMAD diet

Various types of irregular fasting have demonstrated to be powerful in shedding a few pounds of weight. Definitely! It seems like uplifting news. In any case, the OMAD diet isn't suggested by nutritionists as it very well may be hindering for individuals with specific unexpected issues. Moreover, the OMAD diet isn't reasonable for youngsters and grown-ups north of 60. It is not recommendable for people with health conditions such as diabetes and ulcer ***(More on this coming up shortly, keep reading!).

Benefits of the OMAD Diet

◆ ◆ ◆

The point of convergence of the OMAD diet is to lessen your day by day calorie consumption. It's obviously true that expanded calorie utilization is answerable for unnecessary weight gain; to get in shape, you need to chop it down altogether. In any case, it isn't generally easy.

With the OMAD diet, it is very hard to surpass your every day calorie needs, yet that doesn't imply that it is impossible.

Remember: OMAD diet plan isn't really for kids, pregnant or lactating ladies, or when you are on a prescription that requires nourishment for legitimate metabolism.

The advantages of the OMAD diet is that it accompanies appropriate weight the executives, diminished danger of ongoing infections related with exorbitant eating of undesirable food, and worked on metabolic benefits.

When you are battling with getting in shape in spite of eating low carb suppers, possibly all you really want is to launch the weight reduction key arrangement with the impermanent utilization of the OMAD diet plan. It has done some amazing things for many.

Research dated back to 2005 shows that time-confined eating can further develop your body's protection from sickness. The cycle will in general put cells under sure pressure, similarly as weight lifting can cause 'tears' which thus makes the

muscle strands develop back stronger.

OMAD assists with controlling diabetes and improvement in metabolic conditions.

If you are on a tight eating routine timetable that limits eating, then, at that point, OMAD diet plan could be an ideal plan

Other advantages of the OMAD diet include:

⸬ **Saves time and quite economical**

It may sound dubious, yet rehearsing OMAD is to be sure very conservative, and it saves additional time. Envision the time spent planning dinners threefold every day; basically you normal two hours thinking, looking for food things, handling, getting ready, and eating a supper. Keep in mind, you actually need to wash your dishes as well.

If your work schedule is a very tight one or you travel often, or you work in shift, and you can't possibly devote up to 5-6 hours daily preparing and having your meals, then this diet plan could be good for you if you are planning to lose weight.

◢ It encourages healthy eating

Imagine breaking a 23-hour quick with simply an hour to eat, and you can't put together your eating regimen with respect to snacks or any type of low quality nourishment. You can't bear to risk the chance to eat only once in a day by picking unfortunate food sources that will not support you. During the time of quick, you can undoubtedly abandon undesirable food varieties and afterward zeroing in on sound ones that will give you

the genuinely necessary supplement for the day.

◢ It discourages unhealthy lifestyle/addiction

Taking seven jugs of liquor can diminish to only a couple or even none assuming you are earnest with the OMAD diet. During the one hour eating-window period, you can't go with a standard feast with containers of liquor. It could likewise be that you are dependent on eating trashes consistently; you can't have it outside the one-hour eating window period.

Celebrities That Did OMAD Diet

Most occasions, we generally need to hear from our beloved VIPs to know what they are up to as far as the eating regimen way of life and different sorts of stuff that make them look lovable to us on the screen.

Most superstars are at real fault for evaluating a few eating routine choices in the mission to keep or keep up with their body shape.

Now, how about we analyze the big names who have had accomplishment with eating OMAD.

1. Jack Dorsey

This is the most famous and notorious figure on this rundown. Are you acquainted with the name?

Jack Dorsey is the fellow benefactor of perhaps the most involved social medium organization on the planet Twitter.

He uncovered that his single supper, once in 24 hours, comes up during supper hours, and it comprises of protein, green vegetables, and berries (or dull chocolate for dessert).

2. Channing Tatum

Channing Tatum is a Hollywood entertainer with a beguiling build, which makes him a notorious model figure. He centers intensely around the OMAD diet enduring just on Checker burgers for some time prior to traveling into a assortment of a lot better foods.

3. Herschel Walker

Herschel Walker is a resigned professional football player. He has become renowned for his thorough preparing plan, just as the way that he eats once every day. He referenced that he has been participating in the OMAD diet for more than 20 years. In a meeting with the Atlanta Journal-Constitution, he expressed that he eats bunches of bread and veggies. He additionally added that he has ceased from eating red meat for quite a while however surrenders to chicken meat occasionally.

4. Brooke Shields

Brooke Shields is an exceptionally bustling Hollywood entertainer and TV moderator. Her bustling timetable constrained her into the OMAD diet, where she needs to eat once in a day. She likewise focused on that she needed to head to sleep hungry most occasions after a debilitating day.

Apparently, it has truly assisted her with placing in great shape.

5. Nicole Polizzi (Snookie)

Nicole Polizzi, who is prominently known as Snookie, is a television character and an artist. She shared with regards to how her commitment to the OMAD diet contributed essentially to her weight reduction. She likewise focused on that the OMAD diet assisted her with removing her dependence on liquor. Clearly, the eating routine arrangement has assisted her with shedding pounds, however it has likewise kept her from spending a lot on liquor and food.

6. Kohei Uchimura

Kohei Uchimura, a 7-time Olympic medalist is perhaps the best athlete that the world has at any point known. The Japanese revealed in a meeting that one of the key to his prosperity is eating one supper daily. He eats one dinner after his two exercises day by day. He additionally added that he drinks dark espresso before his feast period.

According to Hohei, adaptability is the key as a gymnastic specialist, and it requires being vacant; when unfilled, it is not difficult to move.

7. Hugh Hefner

Hugh Hefner was the organizer of the famous Playboy magazine. As indicated by reports, he had his feast at supper, which is typically sheep cleave and prepared potato. He kicked the bucket at 91.

Others include:

Corey Feldman

Liz Hurley

Pippa Middleton

Megan Fox

And so on.

My Experience with Trying OMAD

◆ ◆ ◆

Before I talk about my involvement in the OMAD diet, I'll start with my involvement in profound fasting. While developing, I was so sluggish with fasting; at whatever point I hear the word 'fasting,' it is then I start to hunger for food.

I was told to continue around 22 hours of quick; it was a strict exercise in any case. It was so intense for me that I turned out to be extremely feeble and exhausted. My dad was practicing OMAD then, and he advised me to start with 12 to 15 hour fast for a start.

Just as in weight lifting, you need to begin slowly. I progressed to 22 hours of quick; along these lines, when I found out about the OMAD diet, I resembled, "Yea, I can do this."

I attempted this number of times, yet the longest fasting streak I had was for seven continuous days. It was very simple, however I was unable to accomplish such a great deal arduous exercises going into the second to last quarter of the fasting period.

Below are my perceptions and conclusions from my experience evaluating the OMAD diet:

It is not a great idea for energy-sapping activities
I love to do some running and furthermore play football inside my area. While on ordinary fasting, I really do well towards these exercises; nonetheless, I am not consistently at my best. Subsequent to participating in these exercises, my longing to eat turns out to be exceptionally serious, and assuming it isn't an ideal opportunity to eat, I should likely sit pausing and trusting that an opportunity to eat comes so quick. Thusly, when I am on the OMAD diet plan, I attempt to avoid brandishing exercises, so I can monitor the little energy I have for other things.

However, it isn't the most ideal same for one of my partners; she doesn't feel the impact however much I do. She can go on the OMAD diet for a month. It is great when you know your cutoff, and making an effort not to strongly overstretch it.

Practicing OMAD doesn't imply that you eat just anything

Yes! The OMAD isn't explicit to a specific kind of supper; it just permits you to eat inside a particular time span. Does it mean you can go all out to eat only any kind of food? No.

When I began the OMAD eating, I was satisfied I could eat unreservedly. In the mean time, I found such a lot of joy in eating nacho, wings, and bourbon, which I understood isn't giving ideal calories to my body needs. For this reason it is crucial to make a decent dinner improved in supplements. Since it is one dinner daily, I attempt to make it an extraordinary one playing hooky of food.

A great way of self-discipline

One thing I like fasting for is that it has helped me assembled a solid demonstration of discipline in such countless parts of my life. I was so much dependent on liquor at

a moment that I barely eat, I ended up being debilitated, and I understood the time had come to abandon this, yet it was troublesome. Since I began rehearsing some time-confined eating, I was giving up steadily. One reason why I took on the OMAD diet is to get me far from jugs of liquor. Presently, in seven days, I don't take up to 3 jugs, and I have started to lose the energy for it. This is something time-confined eating can accomplish for you.

The Downside of the OMAD Diet: Why It Might Not Be Good For You

❖ ❖ ❖

A: "Gracious! I feel mixed up when I don't eat for six hours."

B: "I can go around nine to twelve hours without eating anything, not water; anything over that, I become weak."

C: "I frequently go on three days dry fasting to some degree once in 4 months."

Do you anticipate that A should go on the OMAD diet without disliking it? It could appear to be a capital punishment to them. Notwithstanding, they can start with other less outrageous types of time-confined eating.

Less outrageous variations of time-limited gobbling that permits as long as eight-hour eating window have demonstrated to be compelling in expanding insulin affectability just as contributing monstrously to weight reduction. In the interim, the OMAD diet permits you to eat once every day, which can accompany eating a huge part of food that can trigger the contrary impact of one's intention.

One of the results of the OMAD diet is that it can prompt an exorbitant expansion in hunger, which causes you to gorge at whatever point the time has come to eat, and this can take the muscle versus fat ratio past the level it was before you

left on the eating regimen. At the point when you gorge, this can prompt a flood in insulin level too, and it could prompt you feeling unwell.

Who should say No to the OMAD diet?

The OMAD diet can be adverse and destructive to kids, the old (60+, sometimes, 55+).

- *Children (including teens)*

Children and more seasoned grown-ups need a consistent admission of calories to meet their day by day calorie necessities to keep up with appropriate wellbeing. Having too little calories may <u>compromise the immune system</u> and breakdown muscle mass.

Pregnant and lactating women

No one necessities to let a pregnant lady know that her condition isn't appropriate for any type of fasting. Her hunger for food will in general twofold, so fasting is far removed, essentially for the creating fetus.

On drugs prescription

Since most drugs accompany eating previously or after a feast, then, at that point, it isn't on the right track to be on any type of fasting during this period. Along these lines, such an individual should avoid the OMAD diet.

The results of OMAD diet can include:

- Blood pressure destabilization
- Confusion
- Dehydratio
- n Dizziness
- Low blood sugar
- (Hypoglycemia) Lightheadedness
- Nausea

<u>Reality:</u> As successful as the OMAD diet is, there is no adequate and persuading examination to finish up and suggest the OMAD diet as a legitimate weight reduction diet plan for everyone.

The Consequences of One Meal A

Day: Is The OMAD Diet Good For You?

◆ ◆ ◆

The OMAD diet plan permits you to follow a trained eating plan, you can't modify your planning, and you can adjust your feast type.

No uncertainty that the OMAD diet is unnecessary time-limited eating, and numerous a period, you can feel denied while rehearsing the eating regimen plan. Really powerful, it accompanies its own consequences.

It is feasible to foster more hunger for food in the wake of initiating this arrangement, as there may be an extraordinary change to your metabolic rate. For some, it isn't attainable to get time-limited to food.

Is the OMAD diet healthy?

One thing you want to be aware of the OMAD diet is that it gives your stomach related chemicals, imperative organs, metabolic capacities a break and furthermore diminishes oxidative weight on the body. Better fasting is the point at which you lessen actual pressure joined with taking suppers with fundamental supplements for your body. (More to be talked about on advantages of rehearsing OMAD diet)

The possible consequences of the OMAD diet

Below are a portion of the possible dangers and adverse results related with the OMAD diet.

You could pass up imperative supplements Eating once every day could make you pass up some significant supplements. For this reason it is vital to eat an even dinner at whatever point you are breaking your quick. It is very important.

Increased degree of unfortunate cholesterol Fasting has been related with an increment in LDL cholesterol, which is something contrary to what you are expecting to achieve.

Slowing down of digestion: Practicing time-confined taking care of feast could slow your metabolic rate, and this can likewise trigger undesirable incidental effects, for example, weight gain.

Difficulty in normal or exhausting wearing exercises/undertakings: Imagine somebody having only one dinner daily, they might potentially participate in standard activities, as it tends to be very intense. You can't wear out the food fuel totally on practices just to become unfilled afterward.

The clinical side effects of practicing OMAD diet

The OMAD diet is fit for setting off conditions such as:

- ✓ Low blood sugar
- ✓ Nausea
- ✓ Lightheadedness
- ✓ Blood pressure destabilization
- ✓ Dehydration
- ✓ Dizziness
- ✓ Physical weakness

✓ Extreme yearning or gorge eating

✓ Fatigue

Concern raised over the practice of OMAD

- **Chronic calorie restriction**

The OMAD diet intends to lessen one's calorie admission; notwithstanding, it can bring about hardships in acquiring sufficient calories assuming that eating OMAD is finished quite a while. Albeit constant calorie limitation appears to be helpful in a weight reduction plan, yet it represents a drawn out hazard because of lower resting metabolic rate, which makes it hard to keep up with weight reduction in the long-run.

- **Eating disorders**

If you have a history of an eating disorder in the past, then the OMAD diet might not be too ideal for you since the OMAD diet allows you to eat in an-hour eating window period, which can trigger a serious eating disorder in some individuals.

- **Exercise**

Many individuals think that it is hard to take part in practices while fasting. Assuming you are in this classification, then, at that point, taking the OMAD diet could be truly extreme and challenging.

- **Inadequate protein intake**

The OMAD could advance protein limitation, as it very well may be hard to burn-through up to your every day protein necessity at a time. To this end arranging an even feast is vital.

- **Abdominal discomfort and diarrhea**

Some track down the act of fasting followed by a lot of food very discomforting (stomach distress), and it could even bring about loose bowels. It isn't true with everybody, except it is possible.

Taking medications that require food

Some individuals are on a drawn out medicine of specific medications, which as a rule require taking food previously or subsequent to utilizing it. A portion of these medications are to be taken at least a time or two every day; thusly, the OMAD can't work for this situation. It is smarter to examine with your medical services supplier on the off chance that different options exist; else, the OMAD diet isn't protected, and it isn't for you.

Warning signs! Stop!

It is typical to encounter little appetite and low energy while fasting. However, if you feel unwell, dizzy, overly fatigued, nauseating, or you have other severe side effects, then it is enough to quit or suspend the OMAD fasting plan. Your primary care physician can assist you with working out more limited fasting plans, and possibly assist you with deciding a few changes that could make OMAD an appropriate choice for you in the future.

***

Note: If your one meal a day consists of basically simple carbs, or highly processed fried foods, then you might feel pretty bad afterward. Nonetheless, it doesn't mean you will not get thinner, yet that could be undesirable weight loss.

Frequently Asked Questions on the OMAD Diet

◆ ◆ ◆

Can I eat anything on the OMAD diet?

There is no limitation on the sort of food you ought to devour; the accentuation is on the way that you can eat inside the one-hour eating window, and quick for the following 23 hours. Notwithstanding, it doesn't mean you ought to simply eat anything; you need to repay your framework for starving it for such a long time. Thusly, you ought to guarantee that your eating routine spotlights on supplement rich food varieties that empower you to get an even diet.

I am on the OMAD diet, what would it be advisable for me I eat?

Do not select simply anything you hunger for; you need to gobble beneficial to compensate for the calories you skipped for the duration of the day. Your feast ought to contain solid fats like olive oil, avocado oil, and nuts, just as a decent extent of protein and low-carbs. An assortment of food will be great since our supplement needs are so various, yet you should know what supplement every food in the blend is contributing.

Does OMAD delayed down my metabolism?

In the since a long time ago run, it will in general lower resting metabolic rate, and this can make weight reduction undeniably challenging to keep up with. To this end you should be certain the OMAD diet is appropriate for you prior to digging into it.

Can I drink espresso on the OMAD diet plan?

You can drink without calorie refreshments outside the one-hour eating window. This implies dark espresso and tea are permitted, just as water.

What time is appropriate to take my meal?

It is dependent upon you, yet guarantee it is not even close to your sleep time. Notwithstanding, picking the morning could make you totally drained before nightfall. It suggested taking the supper after your most dynamic time of the day.

I am on the OMAD diet plan, however I am as yet putting on weight, why?

The less food you devour, the less calories you take in, and consequently the more weight that you lose. You may have been gorging throws out after the long quick, and this would bring about you putting on more weight than you would lose.

What occurs in the event that I eat one supper a day?

Practicing the OMAD diet could accompany any of/or the mix of the accompanying conditions:

- Blood pressure destabilization
- Dehydration
- Dizziness
- Low blood sugar
- Lightheadedness
- Nausea

(Note: The incidental effects are not restricted to this list)

How long would it be advisable for me to rehearse OMAD? Assuming that I continue with it for a really long time, will there be a problem?

OMAD is no question a viable weight reduction plan; nonetheless, most wellbeing specialists don't suggest the OMAD diet as a drawn out essential arrangement for weight reduction. There isn't adequate examination/proof to tell how long it is protected to rehearse OMAD. Accordingly it is best it is done on a present moment basis.

I am prepared for OMAD, how would I go about it?

Pick any time that you feel succeeds your most dynamic time. Suppose 3 pm, and afterward you can pick 4 pm-5 pm as your supper period, and be reliable with it from one day to another. While dishing your food, guarantee you utilize one supper size plate, which can be around 10-12 inches width, and try not to have a feast higher than around 3 creeps to stay away from extreme heaps of food.

Key Notes on OMAD diet

- When on the OMAD diet, it is vital to maintain proper hydration. Calorie-free beverages such as black coffee, tea, and water are allowed throughout the day while on the OMAD diet. In other words, you can take these solvents during the period of fasting when you feel dehydrated.
- It is recommended that you remain consistent with your mealtime and ensure you maintain a 23-hour fasting period.
- When fixing a time for the eating window, opt for a time that succeeds your most active time of the day, as this will enable your body to recover from the physical activities.
- Just because people do it doesn't mean it's healthy for you.
- Long-term OMAD is not right for diabetic patients. However short-term OMAD diet plan can be effective but consult your doctor first.

Best Use of OMAD

◆ ◆ ◆

This guidance did not depend on logical proof or verification, however it depends on individual and clinical experience. Persistent utilization of the OMAD diet plan is certifiably not an ideal practice.

If you are attempting the OMAD diet plan, you probably been rehearsing irregular quick preceding giving this a shot. Involving the OMAD diet plan once to threefold in seven days on non-back to back days could be extremely compelling. For example, in the event that you give it a shot for day 1, avoid recently by eating ordinarily, attempt it again on the third day, and skirt the fourth day again.

Day 1-OMAD

Day 2-Lunch and dinner

Day 3-OMAD

Day 4 – Lunch and dinner

Continue with this pattern and perceive how your body responds to it after the initial seven days. If you observe any positive changes with little or no side effects, then it could be your perfect diet plan for weight loss.

However, it is suggested that you stay with a low-carb diet anticipate OMAD days and non-OMAD days. Generally, an all around formed low-carb diet makes the OMAD diet plan simpler as it will in general lessen hunger and cravings.

Below is an illustration of seven days plan utilizing the skipping method:

Day 1: OMAD. Guarantee you are not devouring over your day by day calorie consumption in one supper. Focus on around 30% protein consumption, 30% fat, and around 3% carb. Organic products, vegetables, and entire grains ought to be remembered for your meals.

<u>Day 2: Eat just two suppers with 16:8 time-confined eating</u>. Make an effort not to surpass 1,800 calories from both meals.

<u>Day 3: Repeat Day 1</u>

<u>Day 4: Repeat Day 2</u>

The Bottom Line

◆ ◆ ◆

Eating one feast a day isn't quite so destructive or hazardous as you would might suspect, yet it isn't a great fit for everybody. Nonetheless, it's anything but a prescribed long haul way to deal with losing weight.

From my experience, it was very simple for me since I have been participating in some type of irregular fasting preceding that. You don't need to do OMAD on the grounds that your companion is doing it and it is working for them. Let your body decides whether it is ideal for you. If you attempt this form of time- restricted eating and you are feeling extremely weak or fatigued, then maybe you should consider less restricted one, and when you are used to those, OMAD could be an option for you later on.

Another method of rehearsing the OMAD diet is exchanging the days with a typical eating plan. This implies in about fourteen days; you ought to have around seven days of OMAD, which can in any case be exceptionally powerful. Try not to be too unforgiving with yourself.

You can likewise evaluate OMAD on days when you have a less bustling timetable or days with less proactive tasks. It very well may be successful as well and can assist you with adjusting and acclimate to the eating regimen plan.

When you are on the OMAD diet plan, be careful to adverse consequences, and attempt to cease in the event that you can't adapt, it's anything but a sink or swim issue. You can attempt again

next time.

The way to progress with OMAD is to pay attention to your body

On the following page are the reward wellbeing tips on weight loss...

Healthful Weight Loss Options

◆ ◆ ◆

The OMAD diet is great for the people who are searching for speedy weight reduction arrangements, yet it isn't appropriate for all. There are other more secure and more refreshing strategies to get in shape. You can evaluate the Mediterranean eating routine, and afterward the OMAD diet could be reasonable for you afterward.

In mission of paying special attention to a weight reduction plan, you can likewise consider these options:

Exercising

Exercise is intended to be a lifestyle for everybody. It is significant for sound living. During works out, calories are scorched and delivered as energy.

Along these lines, on the off chance that you are collecting calories from food, you could adjust the impacts by wearing the overabundances out through works out. You can think about a walkout, running, or any type of activity that your solidarity can take.

Regular consultation with related health practitioners

Do not avoid your dietitian assuming you are enthused about shedding pounds. Try not to assume to utilize weight reduction guidance from a companion without examining it with your dietitian or wellness counselor.

Regulating food portion size

It may be troublesome, however it is conceivable. You can do it! Decrease your food
segment size continuously, and keep an eye out for perceptible changes.

Eat a balanced diet

This is vital. A decent eating regimen is the surest wagered to sound living. A fair eating routine energizes all food classes in the proper extent. It is relied upon to zero in additional on products of the soil in a mission to restrict handled food varieties, which are typically one of the offenders behind weight gain and other ongoing illnesses. Beside weight reduction, a fair eating routine works on in general wellbeing and wellbeing.

Say no to late-night meals

One of the potential reasons for exorbitant weight gain and other persistent medical problems are related with eating late around evening time extremely near sleep time. Try not to set up your supper so late that the stretch between your sleep time and supper will be excessively close. Guarantee that you have up to 4 to at least 5 hours stretch between them.

Lastly, make sure to converse with your primary care physician. Your extreme weight gain could be an aftereffect of a basic ailment. Thusly, you want to counsel your primary care physician for appropriate assessment and suggestions.